How to Survive
Measles

A Comprehensive and Easy-to-Follow Guide on How to Prevent, Diagnose, and Treat Measles, With Tips and Advice from Experts and Survivors.

(Things You Must Know)

By
Isabella White

Table of Contents

Foreword_____ 4

Introduction_____ 6

Chapter 1

Understanding Measles_____ 9

A Brief History of Measles_____9

Transmission and Symptoms_____ 12

Complications and Risk Factors_____ 16

Measles in this Modern Era_____ 19

Chapter 2

Preventing Measles Infection_____ 23

Immunization Recommendations_____23

Maintaining Herd Immunity_____ 27

Avoiding Exposure to the Virus_____ 30

Travel Precautions_____ 33

Chapter 3

Diagnosing Measles_____ 36

Recognizing the Signs and Symptoms_____ 36

Distinguishing Measles from Other Rashes____ 39

Diagnostic Testing and Confirmation_____ 44

Reporting and Tracking Measles Cases_____ 47

Chapter 4

Treating Measles_____51

Managing Fever, Discomfort and Dehydration___ 51
Preventing and Treating Complications_____ 55
Supportive Care and Monitoring_____59
Antiviral and Immunoglobulin Therapy_____67

Chapter 5

Caring for Someone with Measles_____72

Isolation Precautions at Home_____ 72
Maintaining Fluid Intake and Nutrition_____ 75
Monitoring the Condition_____ 78
Controlling the Spread of Infection_____82

Chapter 6

Overcoming and Recovering from Measles_ 87

Physical, Cognitive and Social Impacts_____ 87
Rehabilitation and Recuperation_____91
Advice from Measles Survivors_____96

Conclusion_____ 99
Appendix_____102

*Glossary*_____ 102
*References*_____ 106

Foreword

Measles is a highly contagious viral infection that can lead to serious health complications, especially in infants, young children, and immunocompromised individuals. Once common in childhood, measles vaccination programs have dramatically reduced measles cases and deaths worldwide. However, due to vaccine hesitancy and gaps in immunization coverage, measles outbreaks still occur, posing a real threat to public health.

In this comprehensive guide, Dr. Isabella White provides readers with authoritative and practical information on protecting themselves and their families from measles. Based on the most recent scientific evidence and medical experts' insights, the book covers all aspects of measles, from transmission and symptoms to diagnosis, treatment, and prevention. Readers will learn when to seek medical care, how to manage symptoms at home, and what complications to watch out for.

Notably, Dr. White stresses effective prevention through timely vaccination and herd immunity. She provides clear protocols to isolate and care for someone with measles at home, reducing transmission risk. Readers will also gain reassurance and advice from the stories of measles survivors.

This well-researched book, written in an empathetic style, will provide readers with the knowledge and strategies to avoid measles infection. If exposed, readers will know how to mitigate the impacts through early care and treatment. This practical guide is a-must-read for every household, providing the information needed to face the threat of measles confidently. Forearmed with these facts, the readers will be empowered to protect the health of their families.

Dr. Katherine Singh, MD
Pediatric Infectious Disease Specialist;
Seattle Children's Hospital.

Introduction

Measles is one of the most contagious viral diseases known to humankind. It is transmitted via respiratory droplets and aerosols when an infected person coughs or sneezes. The measles virus can linger in the air and on surfaces for 2 hours after contamination. Over 90% of non-immune individuals will contract measles if exposed.

Before the introduction of the measles vaccine in 1963, major epidemics occurred every 2-3 years in the U.S., leading to an estimated 48,000 hospitalizations and 500 deaths annually. Widespread vaccination led to a greater than 99% reduction in measles cases by 2000. However, due to declining immunization rates recently, measles outbreaks have resurfaced as a public health threat.

Measles begins with a high fever, cough, runny nose, sore throat, and red, watery eyes. The hallmark measles rash starts 3-5 days later, spreading from the hairline down the body. While most people recover fully, measles can cause complications like pneumonia, encephalitis, and even death. Permanent vision loss and neurological damage are also possible. There is no specific treatment for measles; care focuses on managing symptoms, preventing complications, and maintaining nutrition.

Individuals and families can protect themselves during outbreaks by understanding measles risks and taking appropriate precautions. This book provides practical, evidence-based guidance on:

- Recognizing signs and seeking prompt diagnosis
- Isolating and caring for someone ill with measles
- Accessing treatment and rehabilitative support
- Avoiding infection through vaccination and behavioral strategies
- Recovering physically and emotionally in the aftermath

This book is intended for anyone who wants to learn more about measles and how to deal with it. Whether you are a patient, a caregiver, a health professional, or a concerned citizen, this book will provide you with the knowledge and skills you need to survive measles and protect yourself and others from this infection.

The best way to use this book is to read it from start to finish, as each chapter builds on the previous one. However, you can skip to the chapters or sections most relevant to your situation or interest. You can also use this book as a reference or a guide whenever you need to refresh your memory or look for specific information.

Forearmed with the knowledge and strategies in the following chapters, readers can survive measles—both figuratively through prevention and literally should exposure occur.

Let us begin building your measles resilience today.

Chapter 1

Understanding Measles

A Brief History of Measles

Measles is one of the oldest and most widespread infectious diseases in human history. It has affected humans for thousands of years and has shaped the course of civilizations, cultures, and societies.

The origin of measles is unclear, but some experts believe it evolved from a virus that infected cattle, called rinderpest, around the 11th or 12th century BCE. The virus then jumped to humans, probably through close contact with domesticated animals. The earliest evidence of measles in humans comes from ancient China, which was described as a disease with fever and rash in the 4th century BCE.

Measles spread rapidly worldwide, along with trade, migration, and conquest. It reached Europe by the 5th century CE and Africa and the Americas by the 15th and 16th centuries CE, respectively. Measles was often fatal, especially among populations that had no previous exposure to or immunity to the virus. It caused massive epidemics and outbreaks, killing millions of people and wiping out entire communities.

Measles also had a significant impact on the history of medicine and science. It stimulated the development of methods to diagnose, prevent, and treat infectious diseases, such as quarantine, isolation, inoculation, and vaccination. The first recorded attempt to prevent measles was in China, where people inhaled the dried crusts of measles lesions to induce immunity. This practice, known as variolation, was later adopted in other parts of the world, such as India, Africa, and Europe.

The first scientific breakthrough in the fight against measles came in the 18th century when the English physician Edward Jenner discovered that cowpox, a mild disease that affected cows, could protect humans from smallpox, a deadly disease related to measles. Jenner's discovery led to the development of the first vaccine, which paved the way for eradicating smallpox and preventing other diseases.

The first vaccine specifically for measles was developed in the 20th century by the American virologists John Enders and Thomas Peebles. They isolated the measles virus from the blood of an infected child in 1954 and used it to create a live-attenuated vaccine, which was tested on humans in 1961. The vaccine proved to be safe and effective, and many countries around the world soon adopted it.

The introduction of the measles vaccine dramatically impacted the global burden of the disease. According to the WHO, between 2000 and 2019, measles vaccination prevented more than 25 million deaths and reduced global measles mortality by 79%. However, despite the availability and affordability of the vaccine, measles remains a significant public health challenge, especially in regions with low vaccination coverage, weak health systems, and humanitarian crises.

Measles is not a disease of the past. It is a present and real threat that can affect anyone, regardless of age, gender, or location. That is why it is important to be informed and prepared to deal with this infection, whether you are a patient, a caregiver, a health professional, or a concerned citizen.

Transmission and Symptoms

Measles is a highly contagious viral infection that can spread easily from person to person. The virus is transmitted through respiratory droplets, such as saliva, mucus, or aerosols, released when an infected person coughs, sneezes or breathes. The virus can also survive on surfaces and objects for up to two hours and can be transferred by touching or sharing items that have been contaminated.

Measles can infect anyone not immune to the virus, either by vaccination or by previous infection. However, some people are more vulnerable to measles and its complications, such as:

- Children under 5 years of age
- Pregnant women

- People with weakened immune systems, such as those with HIV, cancer, or malnutrition,
- People who are unvaccinated or have an incomplete vaccination

The incubation period of measles, the time between exposure to the virus and the onset of symptoms, ranges from 7 to 21 days, with an average of 10 to 14 days. The symptoms of measles usually appear in two phases:

- The first phase, also known as the prodromal phase, lasts 2 to 4 days and is characterized by fever, cough, runny nose, red eyes, and general malaise. Some people may also develop small white spots, called Koplik's spots, inside the mouth, on the inner cheeks, or the gums.
- The second phase, also known as the exanthematous phase, begins around the 3rd to 7th day of the illness and is marked by the appearance of a red, blotchy, and itchy rash that spreads all over the body, starting from the face and neck and then moving to the trunk and limbs. The rash usually lasts 5 to 6 days

and then fades in the same order as it appeared. The fever may also peak during this phase, reaching 40°C (104°F).

The symptoms of measles can vary in severity and duration, depending on the infected person's age, health status, and immune response. Some people may have mild or no symptoms, while others may have severe or life-threatening symptoms. The most common complications of measles include:

- **Pneumonia:** An infection of the lungs that causes difficulty breathing, chest pain, and coughing. Pneumonia is the most common cause of death from measles, especially among young children and adults.

- **Otitis media:** An infection of the middle ear that causes earache, hearing loss, and discharge. Otitis media can lead to permanent hearing impairment or deafness, especially if left untreated.

- **Diarrhea:** A condition that causes loose or watery stools, abdominal cramps, and dehydration. Diarrhea can result in malnutrition, electrolyte imbalance, and shock, especially among children and older people.

- **Encephalitis:** An inflammation of the brain that causes headaches, confusion, seizures, coma, and death. Encephalitis is a severe but rare complication of measles, affecting about 1 in 1000 cases. It can occur during the acute phase of the illness or several weeks or months later due to a delayed immune reaction, known as subacute sclerosing panencephalitis (SSPE).

- Other complications of measles include conjunctivitis, laryngitis, bronchitis, hepatitis, appendicitis, myocarditis, and miscarriage or premature delivery in pregnant women.

Measles is a preventable and treatable disease, but it can also be a deadly and disabling one. That is why it is important to be aware of its transmission and symptoms and to seek medical attention as soon as possible if you suspect that you or someone you know has measles.

Complications and Risk Factors

Measles can cause serious and sometimes fatal complications, especially among children, pregnant women, and people with weakened immune systems. The most common complications of measles include pneumonia, otitis media, diarrhea, and encephalitis. However, measles can also affect other organs and systems of the body, such as the eyes, the ears, the heart, the liver, the appendix, and the nervous system.

Some of the less common but more severe complications of measles are:

- **Blindness** can result from scarring of the cornea, inflammation of the retina, or damage to the optic nerve due to measles infection or vitamin A deficiency. Blindness can affect up to 60,000 people annually, mostly in low- and middle-income countries.
- **Deafness** can result from damage to the inner ear due to a measles infection or otitis media. Deafness can affect up to 30,000 people per

year, mostly in low- and middle-income countries.

- **Cardiomyopathy** is a heart muscle weakening due to measles infection or heart inflammation. Cardiomyopathy can lead to heart failure, arrhythmia, or sudden death.

- **Hepatitis** is a liver inflammation due to measles infection or the toxicity of some drugs used to treat measles. Hepatitis can cause jaundice, liver failure, or cirrhosis.

- **Appendicitis** is an inflammation of the appendix due to measles infection or obstruction of the appendix by fecal matter. Appendicitis can cause abdominal pain, fever, nausea, vomiting, or perforation of the appendix.

- **Subacute sclerosing panencephalitis (SSPE)** is a rare but fatal complication of measles and is caused by a persistent infection of the brain by a mutated form of the measles virus. SSPE can occur several years after the initial measles infection and can cause progressive neurological deterioration, such as cognitive decline, behavioral changes, seizures, coma, and death.

The risk of developing complications from measles depends on several factors, such as:

- **The age of the infected person.** Children under 5 years of age and adults over 20 years of age are more likely to develop complications than older children and young adults.
- **The immune status of the infected person.** People with weakened immune systems, such as those with HIV, cancer, or malnutrition, are more likely to develop complications than people with normal immune systems.
- **The vaccination status of the infected person.** People who are unvaccinated or have incomplete vaccinations are more likely to develop complications than people who are fully vaccinated.
- **The nutritional status of the infected person.** People deficient in vitamin A, iron, or

zinc are more likely to develop complications than those with adequate nutrition.

- **The environmental and social conditions of the infected person.** People living in crowded, unsanitary, or impoverished settings are more likely to develop complications than those living in clean, spacious, or affluent settings.

Measles is a preventable and treatable disease, but it can also be a deadly and disabling one. That is why it is important to be aware of its complications and risk factors and to take preventive and curative measures to avoid or reduce them.

Measles in this Modern Era

Measles is not a disease of the past. It is a present and real threat that can affect anyone, regardless of age, gender, or location. Despite the availability and affordability of a safe and effective vaccine, measles remains a major public health challenge, especially in regions with low vaccination coverage, weak health systems, and humanitarian crises.

According to the World Health Organization (WHO), in 2020, there were more than 22 million cases of measles and over 200,000 deaths globally. Measles outbreaks can occur even in countries with high vaccination coverage due to gaps in immunization, population movement, and misinformation.

The COVID-19 pandemic has also worsened the situation, as it has disrupted the delivery and uptake of routine immunization services, leaving millions of children vulnerable to measles and other vaccine-preventable diseases. In 2020, about 23 million children missed their first dose of the measles vaccine, and more than 94 million children missed their second dose. This has created a large pool of susceptible individuals, increasing the risk of measles transmission and outbreaks.

The global response to measles has been hampered by several challenges, such as:

- Inadequate funding and resources for measles prevention and control, especially in low- and middle-income countries

- Insufficient political commitment and leadership to prioritize and sustain measles elimination and eradication efforts
- Lack of public awareness and trust in the safety and efficacy of the measles vaccine, fueled by misinformation and anti-vaccine movements
- Difficulties in reaching and vaccinating hard-to-reach and marginalized populations, such as those living in remote, conflict-affected, or urban slum areas
- Weak surveillance and laboratory systems are needed to detect and confirm measles cases and outbreaks and monitor the impact of vaccinations.
- Limited capacity and coordination to respond to measles outbreaks, especially in complex and emergency settings

To overcome these challenges and achieve the global goal of eliminating measles by 2030, the WHO and its partners have developed a new Measles and Rubella Elimination Strategy for 2021–2023. The strategy outlines five key objectives:

- Achieve and maintain high and equitable coverage of measles and rubella vaccinations through routine immunization and supplementary immunization activities.
- Identify and close immunity gaps through high-quality surveillance and data analysis.
- Respond rapidly and effectively to measles and rubella outbreaks.
- Strengthen health systems and immunization programs to deliver integrated and people-centered services.
- Mobilize and sustain political commitment, resources, and partnerships for measles and rubella elimination.

The strategy also emphasizes the need to integrate measles and rubella vaccination with other essential health interventions, such as vitamin A supplementation, deworming, and screening for malnutrition, to improve the overall health and well-being of children and communities.

Chapter 2

Preventing Measles Infection

Immunization Recommendations

Immunization is the best way to prevent measles infection and its complications. Immunization involves receiving a vaccine that stimulates the body's immune system to produce antibodies that protect against the disease. The vaccine that protects against measles is called the measles, mumps, and rubella (MMR) vaccine. It also protects against two other diseases: mumps and rubella.

The MMR vaccine is safe, effective, and inexpensive. It is made from weakened or attenuated versions of the viruses that cause measles, mumps, and rubella. The vaccine does not cause the disease, but it may cause mild side effects, such as fever, rash, or swelling at the injection site. These side effects are usually mild and short-lived, and they do not outweigh the benefits of the vaccine.

The MMR vaccine is recommended for all children and adults who do not have evidence of immunity against measles. Evidence of immunity means that you have either:

- *Received two doses of the MMR vaccine or a measles-containing vaccine.*
- *Had a blood test that shows you are immune to measles.*
- *Had measles in the past, confirmed by a doctor.*
- *Were born before 1957 (for adults only).*

The MMR vaccine is given in two doses, separated by at least 28 days. The first dose is usually given at 12 to 15 months of age, and the second dose at 4 to 6 years of age. However, the vaccine can be given earlier or later, depending on the individual's situation and risk of exposure.

Some people may need additional doses of the MMR vaccine, such as:

- Travelers who are going to areas where measles is common or where outbreaks are occurring. They should receive two doses of the MMR vaccine, at least 28 days apart, before departure. Infants 6 to 11 months of age should receive one dose of the MMR vaccine before travel and then two more doses according to the routine schedule.
- Healthcare workers who are in contact with patients who may have measles. They should receive two doses of the MMR vaccine, at least 28 days apart, unless they have evidence of immunity.
- Students at post-high school educational institutions, such as colleges, universities, or vocational schools. They should receive two doses of the MMR vaccine, at least 28 days apart, unless they have evidence of immunity.
- People who have been exposed to measles or who are part of an outbreak. They should

receive one dose of the MMR vaccine as soon as possible unless they have evidence of immunity. This may provide some protection or reduce the severity of the disease.

The MMR vaccine is not recommended for some people, such as:

- People who have a severe allergy to any component of the vaccine, such as gelatin or neomycin
- People who have a weakened immune system, such as those with HIV, cancer, or malnutrition, or those who are taking immunosuppressive drugs
- Pregnant women or women who are planning to become pregnant within 4 weeks of vaccination
- People who have received another live vaccine, such as varicella or yellow fever, within 4 weeks of vaccination
- People who have received a blood transfusion or other blood product within 11 months of vaccination

If you are not sure whether you or your child should receive the MMR vaccine, talk to your healthcare provider. They can help you assess your risk of measles and your eligibility for the vaccine.

Immunization is the best way to prevent measles and protect yourself and others from this serious disease. Make sure you and your family are up to date on your MMR vaccination, and follow the immunization recommendations for your age, health status, and travel plans.

Maintaining Herd Immunity

Maintaining herd immunity is a key strategy to prevent the spread of infectious diseases, such as measles, that can be prevented by vaccination. Herd immunity occurs when a large proportion of a population is immune to a disease, either by vaccination or by natural infection, making it unlikely that the disease will spread from person to person. This also protects those who are not immune, such as infants, pregnant women, or immunocompromised people, who are more vulnerable to the disease and its complications.

The level of herd immunity needed to prevent a disease depends on how contagious the disease is. For measles, which is one of the most contagious diseases, it is estimated that at least 95% of the population needs to be immune to achieve herd immunity. This means that 95 out of 100 people need to have received two doses of the measles vaccine or have had measles in the past and developed natural immunity.

However, maintaining herd immunity is not easy, as many factors can reduce the level of immunity in a population, such as:

- Low vaccination coverage due to lack of access, availability, or affordability of vaccines or due to vaccine hesitancy, refusal, or misinformation
- Population movements, such as migration, travel, or displacement, can introduce new susceptible individuals or new strains of the disease.

- Waning immunity, due to the natural decline of antibodies over time or due to the emergence of new variants of the disease that can evade the existing immunity
- Outbreaks, or epidemics, can overwhelm the health system and the immunization program and expose a large number of people to the disease.

Therefore, to maintain herd immunity, it is important to:

- Ensure high and equitable vaccination coverage, especially among children, who are the main reservoirs and transmitters of measles.
- Monitor and track the immunization status and the disease incidence in the population using reliable surveillance and data systems.
- Respond quickly and effectively to any cases or outbreaks of measles by providing timely diagnosis, treatment, isolation, and contact tracing.

- Educate and engage the public and stakeholders about the benefits and safety of vaccination and address any myths or misconceptions about measles and the vaccine.
- Collaborate and coordinate with other countries and regions to share information and resources and to prevent cross-border transmission of measles.

Maintaining herd immunity is a collective responsibility and a public good, that requires the participation and cooperation of everyone in society.

Avoiding Exposure to the Virus

Measles is a highly contagious viral infection that can easily spread from person to person. The virus is transmitted through respiratory droplets, such as saliva, mucus, or aerosols, released when an infected person coughs, sneezes or breathes. The virus can also survive on surfaces and objects for up to two hours and can be transferred by touching or sharing items that have been contaminated.

To avoid exposure to the virus, you should follow these general guidelines:

- If you have not already done so or if you do not have evidence of immunity, get vaccinated against measles with the measles, mumps, and rubella (MMR) vaccine. The MMR vaccine is safe, effective, and inexpensive. It can protect you from getting sick or developing severe complications from measles. It can also protect others who are not immune, such as infants, pregnant women, or immunocompromised people, by preventing the spread of the disease.

- Avoid contact with people who have measles or who have symptoms of measles, such as fever, cough, runny nose, red eyes, and rash. If you have been in close contact with someone who has measles, follow the quarantine and testing recommendations from your health care provider or local health authority.

- Stay home if you have measles or have symptoms of measles, and isolate yourself from others in your household. Seek medical attention if you have trouble breathing, chest pain, confusion, or other severe or worsening symptoms.

- Wear a mask that covers your mouth and nose when you are in public settings or around people who do not live in your household, especially when you cannot maintain a physical distance of at least 6 feet (about 2 arm lengths) from others. This can help reduce the risk of transmitting or inhaling the virus.

- Wash your hands frequently with soap and water for at least 20 seconds, or use an alcohol-based hand sanitizer that contains at least 60% alcohol, especially before and after touching your face, eating, or using the bathroom. This can help remove or kill the virus from your hands and prevent it from entering your body through your eyes, nose, or mouth.

- Clean and disinfect frequently touched surfaces and objects, such as doorknobs, countertops, keyboards, and phones, using a household cleaner or a diluted bleach solution. This can help eliminate or reduce the virus from the environment and prevent it from being transferred to your hands or other items.

By avoiding exposure to the virus, you can help protect yourself and others from measles and its complications. You can also contribute to the global effort to eliminate this disease by 2030.

Travel Precautions

Traveling can be an exciting and rewarding experience, but it can also expose you to the risk of measles and other infectious diseases. Measles is common in many parts of the world, especially in regions with low vaccination coverage, weak health systems, and humanitarian crises. Travelers who are not immune to measles can get infected and spread the disease to others, both during and after their trip.

To prevent measles infection and transmission while traveling, you should follow these precautions:

- Check your immunization status and get vaccinated if needed. The best way to protect yourself and your loved ones from measles is by getting vaccinated with the measles, mumps, and rubella (MMR) vaccine. You should plan to be fully vaccinated at least two weeks before you depart. If your trip is less than 2 weeks away and you're not protected against measles, you should still get a dose of the MMR vaccine. Infants 6 to 11 months of age should receive one dose of the MMR vaccine before travel and then two more doses according to the routine schedule.

- Check the measles situation at your destination and take extra precautions if needed. You can find the latest information on measles outbreaks and travel health notices on the CDC website or the WHO website. Suppose you are traveling to an area where measles is common or where outbreaks are occurring. In that case, you should avoid crowded and poorly ventilated places, wear a mask, wash your hands frequently, and monitor your health for 3 weeks after you return.

- Seek medical attention if you develop symptoms of measles. If you or your child gets sick with a rash and fever, call your doctor or local health authority. Tell them you traveled abroad and whether you have received the MMR vaccine. They can help you get tested and treated for measles and prevent further transmission to others.

Traveling can be a fun and enriching activity, but it can also pose a risk of measles and other diseases. By following these travel precautions, you can reduce your risk of measles and enjoy your trip safely and healthily.

Chapter 3

Diagnosing Measles

Recognizing the Signs and Symptoms

Measles is a viral infection that causes fever, cough, runny nose, red eyes, and a characteristic rash that spreads all over the body. Measles can also lead to serious complications, such as pneumonia, ear infections, diarrhea, brain inflammation, and even death.

Recognizing the signs and symptoms of measles is important for early diagnosis and treatment, as well as for preventing further transmission to others. The signs and symptoms of measles usually appear in two phases:

- The first phase, also known as the prodromal phase, lasts for 2 to 4 days and is characterized by:
  - Fever, which can range from mild to high and may increase over time.
  - Cough, which can be dry or productive and may worsen over time.
  - Runny nose, which can be clear or thick and may cause sneezing or nasal congestion
  - Red eyes, which can be watery or sensitive to light and may cause itching or burning sensations
  - General malaise, which can include headache, body ache, fatigue, or loss of appetite

Some people may also develop small white spots, called Koplik's spots, inside the mouth, on the inner cheeks, or the gums. These spots are a distinctive sign of measles and usually appear 1 to 2 days before the rash.

- The second phase, also known as the exanthematous phase, begins around the 3rd to 7th day of the illness and is marked by:
  - A rash is the most visible and recognizable symptom of measles. It is red, blotchy, and itchy and spreads all over the body, starting from the face and neck and then moving to the trunk and limbs. The rash usually lasts for 5 to 6 days and then fades in the same order as it appeared.
  - Fever, which may peak during this phase, reaching up to 40°C (104°F).

The signs and symptoms of measles can vary in severity and duration, depending on the infected person's age, health status, and immune response. Some people may have mild or no symptoms at all, while others may have severe or life-threatening symptoms. The most common complications of measles include pneumonia, otitis media, diarrhea, and encephalitis.

Suppose you or your child have any of these signs and symptoms. In that case, you should contact your healthcare provider or local health authority as soon as possible. They can help you confirm the diagnosis of measles and provide you with the appropriate treatment and care.

Distinguishing Measles from Other Rashes

Measles is a viral infection that causes a distinctive red, blotchy, and itchy rash that spreads all over the body. However, other conditions can also cause rashes, such as heat rash, roseola, or allergic reactions. It is important to be able to distinguish measles from other rashes, as they may have different causes, treatments, and complications.

Here are some tips on how to tell the difference between measles and other rashes:

- Look at the timing and pattern of the rash. Measles rash usually appears 3–5 days after the onset of fever, cough, runny nose, red eyes, and white spots in the mouth. The rash starts on the face and neck and then spreads to the rest of the body. The rash lasts for about a week and then fades in the same order as it appeared.

Heat rash, also known as prickly heat or miliaria, usually occurs in hot and humid weather when the sweat glands are blocked and the skin becomes irritated. The rash consists of small, red, and itchy bumps that appear on the neck, chest, back, or groin. The rash may last for a few days and then go away when the skin cools down.

Roseola, also known as sixth disease or exanthem subitum, is a viral infection that affects young children. The rash appears after a high fever that lasts for 3 to 5 days. The rash consists of small, pink, and flat spots that appear on the trunk, arms, and legs. The rash may last for a few hours or days and then disappear without treatment.

Allergic reactions, such as contact dermatitis or hives, can occur when the skin is exposed to something that triggers an immune response, such as a food, a drug, a plant, or an insect bite. The rash can vary in appearance, depending on the type and severity of the reaction. The rash may consist of red, swollen, and itchy patches, blisters, or welts that appear on the area of contact or other parts of the body. The rash may last for a few minutes, hours, or several days, depending on the cause and treatment.

- Look at the other symptoms and signs. Other symptoms, such as high fever, cough, runny nose, red eyes, and white spots in the mouth, often accompany measles. These symptoms usually precede the rash and may persist or worsen during the rash. Measles can also cause serious complications, such as pneumonia, ear infections, diarrhea, brain inflammation, and death.

Heat rash does not usually cause any other symptoms except for mild itching and discomfort. However, heat rash can increase the risk of skin infections if the skin is scratched or damaged. Roseola usually causes a high fever that lasts for 3 to 5 days before the rash appears. The fever may cause seizures, irritability, or lethargy in some children. The rash does not usually cause any other symptoms and does not need any treatment.

Roseola does not usually cause any complications unless the child has a weakened immune system. Allergic reactions can cause a variety of symptoms, depending on the type and severity of the reaction. The symptoms may include itching, swelling, redness, pain, burning, or tingling on the skin or in the mouth, throat, or eyes.

The symptoms may also include sneezing, a runny nose, wheezing, coughing, or difficulty breathing. The symptoms may occur immediately or within a few hours after exposure to the allergen. Allergic reactions can cause serious complications, such as anaphylaxis, which is a life-threatening condition that requires immediate medical attention.

- Seek medical advice. If you or your child have a rash that looks like measles, or if you have been exposed to someone who has measles, you should contact your healthcare provider or local health authority as soon as possible. They can help you confirm the diagnosis of measles and provide you with the appropriate treatment and care.

They can also advise you on how to prevent spreading the disease to others by isolating yourself from others, wearing a mask, and practicing good hygiene. Suppose you or your child have a rash that does not look like measles but is accompanied by other symptoms, such as fever, cough, difficulty breathing, or signs of infection.

In that case, you should also seek medical advice. They can help you identify the cause of the rash and provide you with the appropriate treatment and care. They can also advise you on how to avoid or manage the triggers of the rash, such as heat, allergens, or irritants.

Diagnostic Testing and Confirmation

Measles is a viral infection that can be diagnosed based on its clinical features, such as fever, cough, runny nose, red eyes, white spots in the mouth, and rash. However, these features can also be caused by other conditions, such as roseola, rubella, or allergic reactions. Therefore, it is important to confirm the diagnosis of measles with laboratory tests, especially in cases of doubt, complications, or outbreaks.

Two main types of laboratory tests can be used to confirm measles infection:

- Serological tests detect the presence of antibodies against the measles virus in the blood. Antibodies are proteins that the immune system produces to fight infections. Two types of antibodies can be measured: immunoglobulin M (IgM) and immunoglobulin G (IgG). IgM antibodies appear first, usually within 3 to 4 days after the onset of the rash, and indicate a recent or current infection. IgG antibodies appear later, usually within 2 to 3 weeks after the onset of the rash, and indicate a past or resolved infection. Serological tests can be performed using enzyme-linked immunosorbent assay (ELISA) or immunofluorescence assay (IFA) techniques. Serological tests are useful for confirming individual cases of measles as well as monitoring the immune status and vaccination coverage of a population.

- Virological tests detect the presence of the measles virus or its genetic material in the body fluids or tissues; the measles virus can be isolated from the throat, nose, urine, blood, or cerebrospinal fluid of an infected person using cell culture or animal inoculation techniques. The genetic material of the measles virus can be amplified and identified from the same samples using polymerase chain reaction (PCR) or reverse transcriptase PCR (RT-PCR) techniques. Virological tests can be performed within 7 to 10 days after the onset of the rash and are useful for confirming outbreaks of measles as well as for characterizing the strains of the virus and tracing the sources and routes of transmission.

The choice of the laboratory test depends on the availability, the cost, the timing, and the purpose of the test. In general, serological tests are more widely available and less expensive than virological tests, but they may need help to distinguish between vaccine-induced and natural immunity or between measles and other related diseases. Virological tests are more sensitive and specific than serological tests, but they require more specialized equipment and expertise, and they may not be able to detect the virus in all cases of measles.

The interpretation of the laboratory results should also take into account the clinical features, the vaccination history, and the epidemiological context of the suspected case of measles. A positive result indicates that the person has been infected with the measles virus, either recently or in the past. A negative result indicates that the person has not been infected with the measles virus or that the infection occurred too early or too late for the test to detect it. A doubtful or indeterminate result indicates that the test was inconclusive and that a repeat or a different test may be needed.

Laboratory testing and confirmation are essential for the accurate diagnosis and effective management of measles. They can help to provide appropriate treatment and care, to prevent further transmission and complications, and to monitor and evaluate the impact of vaccination and other prevention and control measures.

Reporting and Tracking Measles Cases

Measles is a notifiable disease, which means that any suspected or confirmed case of measles should be reported to the appropriate health department as soon as possible. Reporting and tracking measles cases are essential for the surveillance and control of the disease, as they can help to:

- Identify and investigate the source and the contacts of the case and provide them with testing, treatment, isolation, or vaccination, as needed.

- Monitor the incidence and trends of the disease and detect any outbreaks or clusters of cases.
- Evaluate the effectiveness and coverage of the vaccination program and identify any gaps or barriers to immunization.
- Provide timely and accurate information and guidance to the public and stakeholders, and address any concerns or misconceptions about the disease or the vaccine.
- Share data and best practices with other countries and regions to support the global effort to eliminate and eradicate measles.

The reporting and tracking of measles cases involve several steps, such as:

- Case detection and notification, which is the process of identifying and reporting any person who has signs and symptoms of measles or who has been exposed to someone who has measles, to the health department. This can be done by health care providers, laboratories, schools, or individuals using standard forms or electronic systems.

- Case investigation and confirmation, which is the process of verifying the diagnosis of measles, involves collecting clinical, epidemiological, and laboratory information from the case and the contacts. Health department staff can use interviews, examinations, tests, and records to do this.

- Case classification and analysis is the process of categorizing the case according to the case definition and analyzing the data to determine the characteristics and risk factors of the case and the contacts. Health department staff can use criteria, algorithms, and software to do this.

- Case response and follow-up, which is the process of providing appropriate interventions and services to the case and the contacts and monitoring their health status and outcomes. This can be done by health department staff in collaboration with healthcare providers, community partners, and other agencies.

The reporting and tracking of measles cases require the coordination and cooperation of various actors and sectors, such as healthcare providers, laboratories, schools, the media, and the public. They also require adherence to ethical and legal principles and standards, such as confidentiality, privacy, consent, and data protection. Reporting and tracking measles cases are vital for accurate diagnosis and effective disease management.

Chapter 4

Treating Measles

Managing Fever, Discomfort and Dehydration

Measles is a viral infection that can cause fever, discomfort, and dehydration, among other symptoms and complications. Fever is the body's natural response to fight the infection, but it can also cause headaches, body aches, fatigue, or a loss of appetite.

Discomfort is the feeling of pain, itching, or irritation caused by the rash, the cough, the runny nose, or the red eyes. Dehydration is the loss of water and electrolytes from the body caused by fever, sweating, diarrhea, or vomiting.

Managing fever, discomfort, and dehydration is important for the recovery and well-being of the person who has measles. It can also help to prevent or reduce the severity of some complications, such as pneumonia, ear infections, or brain inflammation. Here are some tips on how to manage fever, discomfort, and dehydration:

- Drink plenty of fluids, such as water, juice, soup, or oral rehydration solution, to replace the fluids and electrolytes lost from the body. Avoid drinks that contain caffeine, alcohol, or sugar, as they can worsen dehydration or irritate the stomach. Drink at least 8 glasses of fluid per day or more if you have diarrhea or vomiting.

- Acetaminophen (paracetamol) or ibuprofen can lower the fever and relieve pain or inflammation. Follow the dosage and instructions on the label or as prescribed by your doctor. Do not take aspirin, as it can increase the risk of bleeding or Reye's syndrome, a rare but serious condition that affects the liver and the brain.

- Apply cool or wet compresses to the forehead, the neck, or the armpits to reduce body temperature and discomfort. You can also take a lukewarm bath or shower or sponge the body with cool water. Do not use ice or cold water, as they can cause shivering or shock.

- Wear loose and comfortable clothing, preferably made of cotton or other natural fabrics, to allow the skin to breathe and to prevent overheating or irritation. Avoid wearing wool, synthetic, or tight-fitting clothing, as they can trap heat or cause itching or rash.

- Stay in a cool and well-ventilated room, away from direct sunlight or heat sources such as heaters, fireplaces, or stoves. Use a fan or an air conditioner to circulate the air and lower the temperature. Avoid smoking or exposure to smoke, dust, or chemicals, as they can worsen the cough or the red eyes.

- Use a humidifier or vaporizer to add moisture to the air and ease breathing and coughing. You can also inhale steam from a bowl of hot water or a shower or use saline nasal drops or sprays to clear the nasal passages and relieve the runny nose.

- Use artificial tears or eye drops to lubricate and soothe the red eyes. You can also place cold or wet tea bags or cucumber slices over the eyes to reduce the swelling or irritation. Avoid rubbing or scratching the eyes, as they can cause infection or damage. Wear sunglasses or avoid bright lights, as they can hurt the eyes.

- Apply calamine lotion or hydrocortisone cream to the rash to reduce the itching and inflammation. You can also take oatmeal or baking soda baths or apply aloe vera gel or honey to the rash to soothe and heal the skin. Avoid scratching or picking the rash, as these can cause infection or scarring. Cut the nails short or wear gloves to prevent scratching.

Managing fever, discomfort, and dehydration can help to improve the quality of life and the recovery of the person who has measles.

Preventing and Treating Complications

Measles is a viral infection that can cause serious and sometimes fatal complications, especially among children, pregnant women, and people with weakened immune systems. The most common complications of measles include pneumonia, otitis media, diarrhea, and encephalitis. However, measles can also affect other organs and systems of the body, such as the eyes, the ears, the heart, the liver, the appendix, and the nervous system.

Preventing and treating complications of measles is important for the survival and recovery of the person who has measles. It can also help to reduce the burden and cost of the disease on the individual, the family, and society. Here are some tips on how to prevent and treat complications of measles:

- If you have not already done so or if you do not have evidence of immunity, get vaccinated against measles with the measles, mumps, and rubella (MMR) vaccine. The MMR vaccine is the best way to prevent measles and its complications. It can protect you from getting sick or developing severe complications from measles. It can also protect others who are not immune, such as infants, pregnant women, or immunocompromised people, by preventing the spread of the disease.

- Seek medical attention as soon as possible if you have measles or have symptoms of measles, such as fever, cough, runny nose, red eyes, and rash. Your doctor can help you confirm the diagnosis of measles and provide you with the appropriate treatment and care. They can also monitor your condition and check for any signs of complications, such as difficulty breathing, chest pain, confusion, or seizures.

- Acetaminophen (paracetamol) or ibuprofen can lower the fever and relieve pain or inflammation. Follow the dosage and instructions on the label or as prescribed by your doctor. Do not take aspirin, as it can increase the risk of bleeding or Reye's syndrome, a rare but serious condition that affects the liver and the brain.

- Drink plenty of fluids, such as water, juice, soup, or oral rehydration solution, to prevent or treat dehydration. Dehydration can result from fever, sweating, diarrhea, or vomiting. It can also cause malnutrition, electrolyte imbalance, and shock. If you have diarrhea or vomiting, drink at least 8 glasses of fluids per day or more.

- Eat a healthy and balanced diet rich in protein, vitamins, and minerals to boost your immune system and help your body fight the infection. Avoid foods that are spicy, oily, or hard to digest, as they can irritate your stomach or intestines. Eat small and frequent meals, and avoid skipping meals.

- Take vitamin A supplements, as recommended by your doctor. Vitamin A deficiency can increase the risk and severity of measles and its complications, such as blindness, pneumonia, or diarrhea. Vitamin A supplements can help prevent or treat vitamin A deficiency and reduce mortality and morbidity from measles. Vitamin A supplements are especially important for children under 5 years of age, pregnant women, and people with malnutrition or HIV infection.

- Take antibiotics, as prescribed by your doctor, if you have a bacterial infection, such as pneumonia, otitis media, or appendicitis. Antibiotics can help treat the infection and prevent further complications, such as sepsis, abscess, or perforation. Antibiotics are not effective against viral infections, such as measles, and should not be used without a doctor's prescription.

- Get supportive care, such as oxygen therapy, intravenous fluids, or anticonvulsants, if you have severe or life-threatening complications, such as encephalitis, cardiomyopathy, or hepatitis. Supportive care can help stabilize your vital signs, such as blood pressure, heart rate, or oxygen level, and prevent further damage to your organs or systems. Supportive care may require hospitalization and intensive care.

- Follow up with your doctor after you recover from measles to check for any long-term complications, such as subacute sclerosing panencephalitis (SSPE), which is a rare but fatal complication of measles caused by a persistent infection of the brain by a mutated form of the measles virus. SSPE can occur several years after the initial measles infection and can cause progressive neurological deterioration, such as cognitive decline, behavioral changes, seizures, coma, and death.

Preventing and treating complications of measles can help improve the quality of life and recovery of measles patients.

Supportive Care and Monitoring

Measles is a viral infection that can cause mild to severe symptoms and complications, depending on the age, health status, and immune response of the infected person. Most people who have measles recover within 2 to 3 weeks without any specific treatment. However, some people may need supportive care and monitoring to help them cope with the symptoms and complications and to prevent further transmission and infection.

Supportive care is the provision of interventions and services that aim to relieve the symptoms and improve the comfort and well-being of the person who has measles. Supportive care may include:

- Hydration, which is the administration of fluids and electrolytes, either orally or intravenously, to prevent or treat dehydration. Dehydration can result from fever, sweating, diarrhea, or vomiting. It can cause malnutrition, electrolyte imbalance, and shock.
- Nutrition, which is the provision of a healthy and balanced diet rich in protein, vitamins, and minerals to boost the immune system and help the body fight the infection. Nutrition may also include the supplementation of vitamin A, which can reduce the mortality and morbidity from measles, especially among children under

5 years of age, pregnant women, and people with malnutrition or HIV infection.

- Medication, which is the administration of drugs that can lower the fever, relieve the pain or inflammation, treat bacterial infections, or cause seizures. Medication may include acetaminophen (paracetamol) or ibuprofen for fever and pain, antibiotics for pneumonia, otitis media, appendicitis, or anticonvulsants for encephalitis. Medication should be prescribed by a doctor and taken as directed. Aspirin should be avoided, as it can increase the risk of bleeding or Reye's syndrome, a rare but serious condition that affects the liver and the brain.

- Oxygen therapy, which is the delivery of oxygen, either through a mask, a nasal cannula, or a ventilator, to improve breathing and the oxygen level in the blood. Oxygen therapy may be needed for people who have severe pneumonia, cardiomyopathy, or encephalitis and who have difficulty breathing chest pain, or low oxygen saturation.

- Wound care, which is the cleaning and dressing of the skin lesions or ulcers caused by the rash, the scratching, or the secondary infections. Wound care can help prevent infection, scarring, or bleeding and promote healing and recovery.

- Eye care, which is the lubrication and protection of the eyes, uses artificial tears, eye drops, or sunglasses to soothe and prevent further damage to the eyes. Eye care may be needed for people who have conjunctivitis, keratitis, or retinitis and who have redness, swelling, or pain in the eyes.

- Ear care, which is the cleaning and treatment of the ears, uses ear drops, syringes, or tubes to drain the fluid and relieve the pressure in the ears. It may be needed for people with otitis media who have earache, hearing loss, or discharge from the ears.

Monitoring is the observation and measurement of the signs and symptoms, the vital signs, and the laboratory tests to assess the condition and the progress of the person who has measles. Monitoring may include:

- Temperature, which is the measurement of the body heat using a thermometer, to check for fever or hypothermia. Fever is a sign of infection and inflammation and can cause headaches, body aches, fatigue, or a loss of appetite. Hypothermia is a sign of shock or sepsis and can cause confusion, shivering, or unconsciousness.

- Pulse, which is the measurement of the heart rate, is used with a stethoscope, a pulse oximeter, or a monitor to check for tachycardia or bradycardia. Tachycardia is a sign of dehydration, infection, or inflammation and can cause palpitations, chest pain, or shortness of breath. Bradycardia is a sign of brain damage, heart block, or medication overdose and can cause dizziness, fainting, or cardiac arrest.

- Blood pressure, which measures the force of the blood against the walls of the arteries, is measured using a sphygmomanometer, a cuff, or a monitor to check for hypertension or hypotension. Hypertension is a sign of stress, pain, or inflammation and can cause headaches, blurred vision, or strokes. Hypotension is a sign of dehydration, shock, or sepsis and can cause weakness, nausea, or organ failure.

- Respiratory rate, which measures the number of breaths per minute, is measured using a stethoscope, a pulse oximeter, or a monitor to check for tachypnea or bradypnea. Tachypnea is a sign of respiratory distress, infection, or inflammation and can cause coughing, wheezing, or cyanosis. Bradypnea is a sign of brain damage, drug overdose, or sleep apnea and can cause confusion, coma, or death.

- Oxygen saturation, which is the measurement of the percentage of oxygen in the blood using a pulse oximeter or a monitor, is used to check for hypoxemia or hyperoxemia. Hypoxemia is a sign of inadequate oxygen delivery to the tissues and can cause shortness of breath, chest pain, or organ damage. Hyperoxemia is a sign of excessive oxygen delivery to the tissues and can cause headaches, nausea, or seizures.

- Blood glucose, which measures the amount of sugar in the blood, is measured using a glucometer or a monitor to check for hypoglycemia or hyperglycemia. Hypoglycemia is a sign of low blood sugar and can cause sweating, trembling, or confusion. Hyperglycemia is a sign of high blood sugar and can cause thirst, urination, or ketoacidosis.

- Blood count, which is the measurement of the number and type of blood cells, is done using a blood sample and a microscope or a machine to check for anemia, leukocytosis, or thrombocytopenia. Anemia is a sign of low red blood cells and can cause fatigue, pallor, or weakness. Leukocytosis is a sign of high white blood cells and can indicate infection, inflammation, or leukemia. Thrombocytopenia is a sign of low platelets and can cause bleeding, bruising, or petechiae.

- Blood culture, which is the identification of the bacteria or fungi that cause infection in the blood, uses a blood sample and a culture medium or a machine to check for sepsis or bacteremia. Sepsis is a life-threatening condition that occurs when the body's response to infection causes organ dysfunction or failure. Bacteremia is the presence of bacteria in the blood, which can cause fever, chills, or shock.

- Urine analysis, which is the examination of the physical, chemical, and microscopic properties of the urine, uses a urine sample and a dipstick or a machine to check for dehydration, infection, or kidney damage. Dehydration can cause dark, concentrated, or low-volume urine. Infection can cause cloudy, foul-smelling, or bloody urine. Kidney damage can cause protein, glucose, or blood in the urine.

- Chest X-ray, which is the imaging of the lungs and the heart using a machine that emits X-rays to check for pneumonia, pleural effusion, or cardiomegaly. Pneumonia is an infection of the lungs that causes difficulty breathing, chest pain, and coughing. Pleural effusion is the accumulation of fluid in the space between the lungs and the chest wall, which can cause shortness of breath, chest pain, or fever. Cardiomegaly is the enlargement of the heart, which can cause palpitations, chest pain, or heart failure.

Supportive care and monitoring are essential for the treatment and recovery of measles patients. They can help relieve the symptoms and improve their comfort and well-being.

Antiviral and Immunoglobulin Therapy

Measles is a viral infection that can cause mild to severe symptoms and complications, depending on the age, health status, and immune response of the infected person. There is no specific antiviral therapy for measles, as most people recover with supportive care and symptomatic treatment. However, some people may benefit from antiviral and immunoglobulin therapy to prevent or treat severe complications, such as pneumonia, encephalitis, or subacute sclerosing panencephalitis (SSPE).

Antiviral therapy involves the use of drugs that can inhibit or destroy the virus that causes measles. Antiviral therapy may include:

- Ribavirin, which is a nucleoside analog that interferes with the replication of the measles virus. Ribavirin can be given orally or intravenously, and it may reduce the severity and duration of measles symptoms. However, ribavirin has not been proven to prevent or treat measles complications and may cause side effects such as anemia, nausea, or liver toxicity. Ribavirin is not recommended for routine use in measles and should be reserved for severe or complicated cases under the guidance of a specialist.
- Interferon-alpha, which is a cytokine that stimulates the immune system to fight the measles virus. Interferon-alpha can be given intramuscularly or subcutaneously and may prevent or treat measles complications, such as

encephalitis or SSPE. However, interferon-alpha has not been widely studied for measles and may cause side effects such as fever, headache, or injection site reactions. Interferon-alpha is not recommended for routine use in measles and should be reserved for severe or complicated cases under the guidance of a specialist.

Immunoglobulin therapy involves the use of antibodies that can neutralize or eliminate the measles virus. Immunoglobulin therapy may include:

- Measles immunoglobulin (MIG), which is a preparation of antibodies derived from the plasma of donors who have high levels of measles antibodies. MIG can be given intramuscularly or intravenously and may prevent or modify measles infection if given within 6 days of exposure to the virus. MIG is especially indicated for people who are at high risk of severe measles or complications, such as infants, pregnant women, or immunocompromised people who have not been vaccinated or have not developed immunity to measles.

- Intravenous immunoglobulin (IVIG), which is a preparation of antibodies derived from the pooled plasma of many donors. IVIG can be given intravenously and may prevent or treat measles complications, such as encephalitis or SSPE. IVIG may also modulate the immune response and reduce the inflammation caused by the measles virus. IVIG is not recommended for routine use in measles and should be reserved for severe or complicated cases under the guidance of a specialist.

Antiviral and immunoglobulin therapy are not substitutes for vaccination, which is the most effective and safe way to prevent measles and its complications. Antiviral and immunoglobulin therapy are only adjunctive treatments that may be considered for some people who have measles or who are exposed to the virus, depending on their risk factors, clinical condition, and availability of the drugs. Antiviral and immunoglobulin therapy should be used with caution, as they may have side effects, interactions, or contraindications and should be monitored by a healthcare provider.

Chapter 5

Caring for Someone with Measles

Isolation Precautions at Home

Isolation precautions are measures that aim to prevent the transmission of measles from an infected person to others who are not immune. Isolation precautions are especially important for people who have measles or who have symptoms of measles, such as fever, cough, runny nose, red eyes, and rash.

Isolation precautions can help to protect the health and well-being of the person who has measles, as well as their family members, friends, and the community. Isolation precautions at home may include:

- Staying at home and avoiding contact with others until 4 days after the rash appears. This means not going to school, work, or public places, such as shops, parks, or restaurants. It also means having visitors only if they are health care providers or essential services. If you need to leave your home for medical reasons, wear a mask and inform your health care provider or local health authority that you have measles or have symptoms of measles.

- Staying in a separate room and keeping the door closed. If you share a room with others, try to keep a distance of at least 6 feet (about 2 arm lengths) from them, and use a fan or an air conditioner to improve the ventilation. If you share a bathroom with others, try to use it after they have finished, and clean and disinfect it after each use.

- Covering your mouth and nose with a tissue or your elbow when you cough or sneeze and throwing away the used tissue in a lined trash can. Wash your hands with soap and water for at least 20 seconds, or use an alcohol-based hand sanitizer that contains at least 60% alcohol after coughing, sneezing, touching your face, eating, or using the bathroom.

- Not sharing personal items, such as cutlery, cups, towels, clothes, or bedding, with others. Wash your items separately from others, using hot water and detergent, and dry them thoroughly. Clean and disinfect frequently touched surfaces and objects, such as doorknobs, countertops, keyboards, and phones, using a household cleaner or a diluted bleach solution.

- Follow the advice of your healthcare provider or local health authority on how to monitor your condition and check for any signs of complications, such as difficulty breathing, chest pain, confusion, or seizures. Seek medical attention if you have any of these signs or symptoms or if your condition worsens. Inform your healthcare provider or local health authority that you have measles or have symptoms of measles before you visit them or call an ambulance.

Isolation precautions at home are essential for the prevention and control of measles. They can help reduce the risk of transmission and infection and improve the recovery and quality of life of the person who has measles.

Maintaining Fluid Intake and Nutrition

Measles is a viral infection that can cause fever, rash, cough, runny nose, and red eyes, among other symptoms and complications. Measles can also affect the appetite and digestion of the person who has measles and cause dehydration, malnutrition, or weight loss.

Maintaining fluid intake and nutrition is important for the recovery and well-being of the person who has measles. It can also help to prevent or reduce the severity of some complications, such as diarrhea, pneumonia, or encephalitis. Here are some tips on how to maintain fluid intake and nutrition:

- Drink plenty of fluids, such as water, juice, soup, or oral rehydration solution, to replace the fluids and electrolytes lost from the body.

Dehydration can result from fever, sweating, diarrhea, or vomiting. It can cause malnutrition, electrolyte imbalance, and shock. Drink at least 8 glasses of fluids per day or more if you have diarrhea or vomiting. Avoid drinks that contain caffeine, alcohol, or sugar, as they can worsen dehydration or irritate the stomach.

- Eat a healthy and balanced diet rich in protein, vitamins, and minerals to boost your immune system and help your body fight the infection. Protein can help repair the tissues and organs damaged by the virus. Vitamins and minerals can help prevent or treat vitamin A deficiency, which can increase the risk and severity of measles and its complications, such as blindness, pneumonia, or diarrhea. Eat foods that are easy to digest, such as rice, bread, pasta, potatoes, bananas, applesauce, or yogurt. Avoid foods that are spicy, oily, or hard to digest, such as fried foods, beans, or dairy products. Eat small and frequent meals, and avoid skipping meals.

- Take vitamin A supplements, as recommended by your doctor. Vitamin A deficiency can increase the risk and severity of measles and its complications, especially among children under 5 years of age, pregnant women, and people with malnutrition or HIV infection. Vitamin A supplements can help prevent or treat vitamin A deficiency and reduce mortality and morbidity from measles. Vitamin A supplements are usually given in two doses, separated by 24 hours, and should be taken with food or milk to avoid nausea or vomiting.

- Take multivitamin supplements, as recommended by your doctor. Multivitamin supplements can help provide additional vitamins and minerals that may be lacking in your diet due to reduced appetite or digestion problems. Multivitamin supplements can help improve your energy and immunity and prevent or treat deficiencies that may worsen your condition. Multivitamin supplements should be taken according to the dosage and the instructions on the label or as prescribed by your doctor.

- Seek medical advice if you have trouble eating or drinking or if you have signs of dehydration or malnutrition, such as dry mouth, sunken eyes, low urine output, dizziness, weakness, or weight loss. Your doctor can help you assess your nutritional status and your fluid intake and provide you with the appropriate treatment and care. They can also advise you on how to modify your diet and fluid intake according to your needs and preferences.

Maintaining fluid intake and nutrition can help to improve the quality of life and recovery of people with measles.

Monitoring the Condition

Monitoring the condition is the process of observing and measuring the signs and symptoms, the vital signs, and the laboratory tests to assess the condition and the progress of the person who has measles. Monitoring the condition can help to:

- Detect and treat any complications, such as pneumonia, ear infections, diarrhea, or brain inflammation that may arise during the course of the disease.

- Evaluate the response and effectiveness of the treatment and supportive care, such as hydration, nutrition, medication, or oxygen therapy, given to the person who has measles.

- Provide timely and accurate information and feedback to the person who has measles, their family members, and their healthcare providers about their health status and their recovery.

- Prevent further transmission and infection by isolating the person who has measles until they are no longer contagious and by vaccinating or quarantining their contacts who are not immune to measles.

Monitoring the condition may involve several steps, such as:

- Checking the signs and symptoms, such as fever, rash, cough, runny nose, and red eyes, that are characteristic of measles and noting their onset, duration, severity, and frequency. The signs and symptoms of measles usually appear 10 to 14 days after exposure to the virus and last for about 2 to 3 weeks. The rash is the most visible and recognizable symptom and usually appears 3–5 days after the onset of the fever, starting from the face and neck and then spreading to the rest of the body. The rash lasts for about a week and then fades in the same order as it appeared.

- Measuring the vital signs, such as temperature, pulse, blood pressure, respiratory rate, and oxygen saturation, that reflect the functioning of the body's systems and organs. The vital signs can be measured using various devices, such as a thermometer, a stethoscope, a sphygmomanometer, a pulse oximeter, or a monitor. The vital signs can indicate the presence and severity of infection, inflammation, dehydration, shock, or organ damage and can guide treatment and supportive care.

- Performing laboratory tests, such as a blood count, blood culture, urine analysis, or chest X-ray, can confirm the diagnosis of measles and detect any complications, such as anemia, sepsis, kidney damage, or pneumonia. The laboratory tests can be performed using various samples, such as blood, urine, or sputum, and various techniques, such as microscopy, culture, or imaging. The laboratory tests can provide objective and quantitative data and can monitor the response and effectiveness of the treatment and supportive care.

The frequency and intensity of monitoring the condition may vary depending on the age, health status, and immune response of the person who has measles, as well as the availability and accessibility of the resources and services. In general, monitoring the condition should be done at least once a day or more often if the condition worsens or changes.

Monitoring the condition should be done by a health care provider or by a trained and supervised family member or caregiver who can record and report the results and act accordingly. Monitoring the condition is essential for the treatment and recovery of the person who has measles.

Controlling the Spread of Infection

Measles is a highly contagious viral infection that can spread easily from person to person through respiratory droplets, such as saliva, mucus, or aerosols, that are released when an infected person coughs, sneezes or breathes. Measles can also survive on surfaces and objects for up to two hours and can be transferred by touching or sharing items that have been contaminated.

Controlling the spread of infection is important for the prevention and control of measles, as it can help to protect the health and well-being of the person who has measles, as well as their family members, friends, and the community. Controlling the spread of infection can also contribute to the global effort to eliminate and eradicate measles by stopping the transmission and circulation of the virus. Controlling the spread of infection may include:

- Vaccination, which is the administration of the measles, mumps, and rubella (MMR) vaccine, induces immunity against the measles virus. Vaccination is the most effective and safe way to prevent measles and its complications. Vaccination can protect the person who receives the vaccine, as well as others who are not immune, such as infants, pregnant women, or immunocompromised people, by preventing the spread of the disease. Vaccination should be given to all children at 12 to 15 months of age and again at 4 to 6 years of age or as recommended by the local immunization schedule. Vaccination should also be given to adults who have not been vaccinated or have not developed immunity to measles, especially if they are traveling to or living in areas where measles is common or where outbreaks are occurring.

- Isolation, which is the separation of the person who has measles or who has symptoms of measles from others who are not immune, until they are no longer contagious. Isolation can help prevent the exposure and infection of others and reduce the risk of transmission and outbreaks. Isolation should be done at home or in a health care facility, depending on the condition and the preference of the person who has measles. Isolation should last for at least 4 days after the rash appears or as advised by the health care provider or local health authority.

- Quarantine, which is the restriction of the movement and contact of people who have been exposed to the measles virus but who do not have symptoms of measles until they are no longer at risk of developing or spreading the disease. Quarantine can help to identify and monitor the contacts of the person who has measles and to provide them with testing, treatment, isolation, or vaccination, as needed. Quarantine should be done at home or in a designated facility, depending on the risk and the preference of the contacts. Quarantine should last for at least 21 days after the last exposure to the virus or as advised by the health care provider or local health authority.

- Hygiene, which is the practice of maintaining cleanliness and sanitation to prevent or reduce the transmission of the measles virus. Hygiene can help to eliminate or reduce the virus from the environment and personal items and prevent it from entering the body through the eyes, nose, or mouth. Hygiene may include:
    - Washing hands frequently with soap and water for at least 20 seconds or using an alcohol-based hand sanitizer that contains at least 60% alcohol, especially before and after touching the face, eating, or using the bathroom.
    - Covering the mouth and nose with a tissue or the elbow when coughing or sneezing and throwing away the used tissue in a lined trash can.
    - Wearing a mask that covers the mouth and nose when in public settings or around people who are not immune, especially when physical distancing of at least 6 feet (about 2 arm lengths) from others is not possible.

- ○ Cleaning and disinfecting frequently touched surfaces and objects, such as doorknobs, countertops, keyboards, and phones, using a household cleaner or a diluted bleach solution.
- ○ Do not share personal items such as cutlery, cups, towels, clothes, or bedding with others.

Controlling the spread of infection is vital for the prevention and control of measles. It can help to protect the health and well-being of the person who has measles, as well as their family members, friends, and the community. It can also help achieve the global goal of eliminating and eradicating this disease by 2030.

Chapter 6

Overcoming and Recovering from Measles

Physical, Cognitive and Social Impacts

Measles is a viral infection that can cause mild to severe symptoms and complications, such as fever, rash, cough, runny nose, red eyes, pneumonia, ear infections, diarrhea, brain inflammation, and death. Measles can also have physical, cognitive, and social impacts on the person who has measles, as well as their family members, friends, and the community.

Physical impacts are the effects of measles on the body and its functions, such as:

- Skin lesions or scars, which can result from the rash, scratching, or secondary infections, can affect the appearance and self-esteem of the person who has measles.

- Vision loss or blindness, which can result from eye infections or inflammation, such as conjunctivitis, keratitis, or retinitis, can affect the daily activities and quality of life of a person who has measles.

- Hearing loss or deafness, which can result from the infection or the inflammation of the ears, such as otitis media, can affect the communication and social skills of the person who has measles.

- Organ damage or failure, which can result from the infection or the inflammation of the lungs, the heart, the liver, the kidneys, or the brain, such as pneumonia, cardiomyopathy, hepatitis, nephritis, or encephalitis, can affect the health and the survival of the person who has measles.

- Growth retardation or stunting, which can result from the malnutrition or vitamin A deficiency caused by the measles infection, can affect the physical and mental development of the person who has measles, especially children.

- Death, which can result from the severe or life-threatening complications of measles, such as sepsis, shock, or subacute sclerosing panencephalitis (SSPE), can affect the life expectancy and mortality rate of the person who has measles, as well as their family members, friends, and the community.

Cognitive impacts are the effects of measles on the brain and its functions, such as:

- Memory loss or impairment, which can result from an infection or inflammation of the brain, such as encephalitis or SSPE, can affect the learning and recall of a person who has measles.
- Cognitive decline or dementia, which can result from brain infections or inflammation, such as encephalitis or SSPE, can affect the reasoning and judgment of a person who has measles.
- Behavioral changes or disorders that can result from the infection or the inflammation of the

brain, such as encephalitis or SSPE, can affect the mood and personality of the person who has measles.

- Seizures or epilepsy, which can result from an infection or inflammation of the brain, such as encephalitis or SSPE, can affect the electrical activity and coordination of the brain and body of a person who has measles.

- Coma, or vegetative state, which can result from an infection or inflammation of the brain, such as encephalitis or SSPE, and can affect the consciousness and awareness of the person who has measles.

Social impacts are the effects of measles on the relationships and interactions of the person who has measles with their family members, friends, and the community, such as:

- Isolation or stigma, which can result from the separation or discrimination of the person who has measles due to fear or misunderstanding of the disease or the vaccine, can affect the emotional and social well-being of the person who has measles.

- Education or work loss, which can result from the absence or impairment of the person who has measles due to the illness or complications, can affect the academic and economic opportunities and outcomes of the person who has measles.

- Health care or social costs, which can result from the treatment or supportive care of the person who has measles or the prevention or control measures of the disease, such as vaccination, isolation, or quarantine, can affect the financial and social resources and services of the person who has measles, as well as their family members, friends, and the community.

Rehabilitation and Recuperation

Rehabilitation and recuperation are the processes of restoring and improving the physical, cognitive, and social functions and well-being of the person who has measles after they have overcome the acute phase of the disease. Rehabilitation and recuperation can help to:

- Heal and prevent the scars, vision loss, hearing loss, or organ damage that may result from the measles infection or its complications.
- Enhance and maintain memory, cognition, behavior, or mood that may be affected by the measles infection or its complications.
- Reintegrate and reconnect with the family, friends, and the community that may have been isolated or stigmatized due to the measles infection or its vaccine.
- Resume and succeed in education, work, or social activities that may have been interrupted or impaired due to the measles infection or its complications.
- Reduce and manage the health care or social costs that may have been incurred due to the measles infection or its treatment and prevention.

Rehabilitation and recuperation may involve several steps, such as:

- Physical therapy, which is the use of exercises, massage, heat, or cold to improve the strength, flexibility, or mobility of the muscles, joints, or limbs that may have been weakened or injured by the measles infection or its complications
- Occupational therapy, which is the use of activities, devices, or adaptations to improve the skills, abilities, or independence of the person who has measles in performing their daily tasks, such as dressing, eating, or bathing,
- Speech therapy, which is the use of techniques, exercises, or devices to improve communication, language, or swallowing of the person who has measles, may have been affected by hearing loss, brain damage, or throat infection caused by the measles infection or its complications.
- Vision therapy, which is the use of exercises, lenses, or devices to improve the sight, eye movement, or eye coordination of a person who has measles, may have been impaired by vision loss, eye infection, or eye inflammation caused by the measles infection or its complications.

- Psychological therapy, which is the use of counseling, medication, or relaxation to improve the mental health, emotional stability, or coping skills of the person who has measles, may have been disturbed by the stress, trauma, or stigma caused by the measles infection or its vaccine.

- Social support, which is the provision of information, guidance, or assistance to the person who has measles and their family members, friends, or caregivers by healthcare providers, community workers, or peer groups to help them deal with the challenges, needs, or expectations that may arise from the measles infection or its recovery.

- Educational or vocational training, which is the provision of learning, coaching, or mentoring to the person who has measles and their teachers, employers, or colleagues by educators, trainers, or counselors to help them resume, continue, or excel in their academic or professional goals that may have been delayed, disrupted, or affected by the measles infection or its recovery

The duration and intensity of rehabilitation and recuperation may vary depending on the age, health status, and immune response of the person who has measles, as well as the severity and type of the measles infection or its complications.

In general, rehabilitation and recuperation should start as soon as possible, after the person who has measles has recovered from the acute phase of the disease, and should last until the person who has measles has achieved their optimal level of functioning and well-being. Rehabilitation and recuperation should be done by a multidisciplinary team of healthcare providers in collaboration with the person who has measles and their family members, friends, or caregivers.

Rehabilitation and recuperation are essential for the recovery and well-being of a person who has measles. They can help to heal and prevent the physical, cognitive, and social impacts of measles and to improve the quality of life and satisfaction of the person who has measles. They can also help to prevent or reduce the recurrence or transmission of measles by ensuring the completion and maintenance of vaccination and prevention measures.

Advice from Measles Survivors

Recovering from measles can be challenging, but first-hand experiences and wisdom from survivors can provide both practical guidance and emotional support.

Ryan's Story

Ryan was 7 years old when he developed measles shortly before the school year started. He suffered from a high fever, cough, conjunctivitis, and a telltale red, blotchy rash. Although he recovered from the acute illness, Ryan struggled with fatigue, muscle weakness, and memory problems that made school difficult when he returned. With time and support, his health and academic performance improved. Ryan says:

"My advice is to be patient with yourself during recovery; rebuilding your strength takes time. Accept help from family and friends when needed. Set small goals each day and recognize your progress."

Alicia's Experience

As a 24-year-old new mom, Alicia was looking forward to sharing all of her son's first milestones. When they both caught measles from an outbreak at a children's play group, she was terrified. While her son recovered quickly, Alicia suffered pneumonia as a complication, requiring hospitalization. She explains:

"Don't lose hope; even if you have a major setback, healing is possible. Celebrate every step forward. Connect with other survivors who understand what you're going through."

Jamil's Story

Jamil contracted measles at age 5 before the vaccine was available. Now in his 60s, he still has vision impairment from the infection. He says:

"My eyesight is damaged, but I have adapted and live a full life. Advocate for yourself and seek out

rehab services. There are technological tools that can help you adjust."

These inspiring individuals exemplify the resilience and optimism of measles survivors. Their stories offer motivation, reassurance, and guidance for others on the path to recovery.

Conclusion

Measles is an extremely contagious viral disease that can lead to serious complications but is also one that can be effectively prevented and treated. Through vaccination, isolation precautions, supportive medical care, and rehabilitation, most people can fully recover from measles.

In this book, we have covered all aspects of measles, from understanding its history, transmission, and symptoms to diagnosis, treatment, prevention, and recovery. By learning to recognize the signs of measles early, readers can seek prompt medical care and diagnosis, initiating treatment to manage symptoms and prevent progression to more dangerous complications.

Prevention is always better than cure. I encourage readers to ensure they and their families receive the full 2-dose MMR vaccine schedule, which provides long-lasting protection against measles infection. Maintaining herd immunity through high vaccination rates in the community is also critical to stopping the spread of measles.

If exposed to measles, readers now have practical guidance on isolating and caring for someone infected at home. Following the protocols for treatment, monitoring, and managing fever, fluids, and nutrition will aid recovery until the infection passes. The precautions detailed will also help limit transmission to others.

While measles can be serious and frightening, education and preparation take away its power. Armed with the knowledge in this guide, readers can face the threat of measles with confidence in their ability to protect themselves and their families. By working together, we can overcome measles and look forward to a future free from this dangerous but preventable disease.

This book has helped you gain a better understanding and awareness of measles and how to prevent, diagnose, and treat it, with tips and advice from experts and survivors. I also hope that this book has inspired and motivated you to overcome and recover from measles and to resume and succeed in your life goals and aspirations.

Thank you for reading this book, and I wish you all the best in your journey of surviving measles.

Please share your thoughts and opinions about this book by leaving a comment and rating it as well.

Appendix

This appendix contains additional information and resources that may be useful to the readers of this book.

Glossary

This glossary defines some of the terms and acronyms that are used in this book.

- **Antibodies:** Proteins that are produced by the immune system to fight and neutralize foreign substances, such as viruses or bacteria.
- **Antiviral therapy:** The use of drugs that can inhibit or destroy the virus that causes measles.
- **CDC:** Centers for Disease Control and Prevention, a national public health agency in the United States that provides information

and guidance on various diseases and health issues, including measles.

- **Complications:** The secondary or additional problems that may arise from the measles infection, such as pneumonia, ear infections, diarrhea, or brain inflammation.

- **Encephalitis:** The infection or inflammation of the brain, which can cause headache, confusion, seizures, coma, or death.

- **Immunoglobulin therapy:** The use of antibodies that can neutralize or eliminate the measles virus.

- **Immune system:** The system of the body that defends against foreign substances, such as viruses or bacteria, and produces antibodies and immune cells to fight them.

- **Immunization:** The process of inducing immunity against a disease by exposing the body to a weakened or killed form of the disease-causing agent, such as a vaccine.

- **Incubation period:** The period of time between the exposure to the measles virus and the appearance of the first symptoms, which is usually 10 to 14 days.

- **MIG:** Measles immunoglobulin, a preparation of antibodies derived from the plasma of donors who have high levels of measles antibodies.

- **MMR:** Measles, mumps, and rubella, a combined vaccine that protects against three diseases: measles, mumps, and rubella.

- **Mortality:** The number or rate of deaths caused by a disease, such as measles.

- **Morbidity:** The number or rate of cases or complications caused by a disease, such as measles.

- **NHS:** National Health Service, a public health system in the United Kingdom that provides free or subsidized health care services, including vaccination and treatment for measles.

- **Otitis media:** The infection or inflammation of the middle ear, which can cause earache, hearing loss, or discharge from the ear.

- **Pneumonia:** The infection or inflammation of the lungs, which can cause difficulty breathing, chest pain, or coughing.

- **Quarantine:** The restriction of the movement and contact of the people who have been exposed to the measles virus but who do not have symptoms of measles until they are no longer at risk of developing or spreading the disease.

- **Rash:** The red, itchy, or bumpy skin lesions that are caused by the measles virus and that usually appear 3–5 days after the onset of the fever, starting from the face and neck and then spreading to the rest of the body.

- **SSPE:** Subacute sclerosing panencephalitis, a rare but fatal complication of measles, is caused by a persistent infection of the brain by a mutated form of the measles virus, which can cause progressive neurological deterioration, such as cognitive decline, behavioral changes, seizures, coma, and death.

- **Vaccine:** A preparation of a weakened or killed form of a disease-causing agent, such as a virus or a bacterium, that is administered to induce immunity against the disease.

- **WHO:** World Health Organization is a specialized agency of the United Nations that is responsible for international public health and that provides information and guidance on various diseases and health issues, including measles.

References

This section lists some of the sources and references that were used or cited in this book.

- Measles - World Health Organization (WHO) (https://www.who.int/news-room/fact-sheets/detail/measles).
- Measles | CDC (https://www.cdc.gov/measles/index.html).
- Measles - NHS (https://www.nhs.uk/conditions/measles/).
- Measles - Mayo Clinic (https://www.mayoclinic.org/diseases-conditions/measles/symptoms-causes/syc-20374857)

- Measles - Diagnosis & treatment - Mayo Clinic (https://www.mayoclinic.org/diseases-conditions/measles/diagnosis-treatment/drc-20374862).
- Measles - Treatment - NHS (https://www.nhs.uk/conditions/measles/treatment/).
- Measles: Information for Public Health Professionals | CDC (https://www.cdc.gov/measles/hcp/index.html).
- National measles guidelines - GOV.UK (https://www.gov.uk/government/publications/measles-guidance-for-health-professionals).
- Healthcare Facility Infection Control Recommendations for Suspect Measles Patients (https://www.cdc.gov/measles/hcp/infection-control.html).
- Guidelines for Measles Quarantine/Isolation/Furlough - TN.gov (https://www.tn.gov/content/dam/tn/health/

documents/Measles_Quarantine_Guidelines.p
df).

- Measles survivor: 'I was on fire for seven days'
  (https://www.bbc.com/news/health-47940710
).
- Measles survivor: 'I was so weak I couldn't even
  sit   up'
  (https://www.bbc.com/news/health-47933511)
- Measles survivor: 'I wish I had been vaccinated'
  (https://www.bbc.com/news/health-47946065
).
- Measles: symptoms, diagnosis, complications,
  and   treatment   (factsheet)
  (https://www.health.gov.au/resources/publica
  tions/measles-symptoms-diagnosis-complicati
  ons-and-treatment-factsheet).
- Rehabilitation - World Health Organization
  (WHO)
  (https://www.who.int/news-room/fact-sheets/
  detail/rehabilitation).